Table of Contents

Copyright Notice 4
Thank You North Cross Hospital 5
How it All Began 6
My First Major Surgery 7
How it All Went All Wrong 9
Post-Hysterectomy Experience 11
An Emergency Colostomy Surgery 14
A Colostomy, What's That? 18
I Was in Denial 20
Some Good News - My Colostomy was Reversible 22
Physical and Emotional Recovery 24
7 Reasons Why You May Need a Colostomy Surgical Procedure 27
    1. Diverticulitis 28
    2. Crohn's Disease 29
    3. Cancer of the Bowels 30
    4. Obstruction of the Bowels 31
    5. Trauma and Injury 32
    6. An Emergency Situation 32
    7. Bowel Incontinence 34
What to Expect After the Procedure? 35
Coping with My Emotional State after Colostomy Surgery 38
How it Affects Us Emotionally 40
Help and Support for Ostomates 42
The Importance of Making Emotional Progress 44

Don't Be a Slave to Your Feelings	46
My Colostomy Food and Diet Tips	49
Consumption	52
Fibre intake	52
Mastication	53
J Pouch diet	54
What to avoid	54
Fluids	55
Beef and poultry	55
Food and Drinks Guide	56
J Pouch Diet	58
Useful Tips	59
How I Coped with Wearing Bags and Managing a Stoma	60
The First Few Weeks at Home	61
Eating and General Diet	62
Clothing	63
Sleep	64
Partying and Socialising	65
Travelling	67
Major Challenges I Faced Wearing Colostomy Bags	69
Back to My Regular Lifestyle with my Colostomy	71
How I Kept My Stoma Clean, to Avoid Infection	74
How to Clean a Stoma	75
Supplies Required to Keep a Stoma Clean	79
Tips	82
Problems to Expect as an Ostomate	84
Flatulence	85

- Loose/Watery Stool 87
- Bag Leaks 89
- Discomfort in the Rectum 91
- Faceplate Water Absorption 92
- Pancaking (or Patty-caking) 93
- Bag 'Blowouts' 96

Colostomy Reversal One Year After 103
- How Long Does It Take to Fully Recover? 108
- Post-Surgery Monitoring 109
- Recent Studies on Temporary Colostomy Patients 109

My Inspiration 111

Copyright Notice

Copyright © 2020 Alobeda S.

(Portions from my Copyright © 2010, 2015 AloBeDa)

All rights reserved.

Any redistribution or reproduction of part or all of the contents in any form is prohibited.

You may not distribute or commercially exploit the content, nor may you transmit it or store it in any other website or other form of electronic retrieval system, except by reviewers who may quote brief passages in a review. It is prohibited to photocopy, record, or infringe in any other form using electronic or mechanical methods.

Thank You North Cross Hospital

I wish to, once again, thank the North Cross Hospital in Wolverhampton, my surgeon, Mr G. Williams aka 'Mr Bean', the kind doctors on ward rounds, my Stoma Nurse, and all the kind and lovely nurses who took great care of me while I was a colostomy patient in their hospital.

I can never stop being grateful.

How it All Began

When I was eighteen, I woke up one morning with excruciating stomach pains and within a few hours, I was in the hospital. Diagnosis showed I had endometriosis. That perhaps explained why I always had painful periods and cramping before the onset of my periods and extended several days into it.

I spent a couple of days and was subsequently discharged. I was placed on some form of medication. Case closed, or so I thought. Ten years down the line, I discovered that I had difficulties conceiving, after a series of doctors' visits and tests, I found that I had fibroids.

And so, the horrible 'journey' began.

My First Major Surgery

The first surgical procedure I had was a myomectomy, an operation involving the removal of uterine fibroids. I was in my late twenties. My surgeon told me that he successfully removed some, but the tinier fibroids were hard to remove, so he left them in.

Finally, I heaved a sigh of relief that it was all over, but it wasn't. I still didn't get pregnant. Then the fibroids started to grow back. Did I hear that an 'idle' womb breeds fibroids? I think I did, somewhere.

It was recommended that I shrink them with injections, but they never helped beyond a few months, so, I had to have a second myomectomy. However, by the time I dared to undergo surgery again, the fibroids had become so large, they weighed close to 5 kilos. It became an issue to remove them or squeeze your other organs to 'death'. Many people thought I was heavily pregnant; that's how massive they were. They just had to be removed.

How it All Went All Wrong

I checked into a private hospital in Wolverhampton in the UK. I was booked to undergo a myomectomy, stay in a hospital for a maximum of 7 to 10 days, heal well, and continue with my life. I was tired of walking around looking like a seven months pregnant woman.

During surgery, it was discovered that my uterus had adhered (gummed was the word they used) to parts of my digestive organs. Reasons adduced? The sheer size and rate of growth of my uterine fibroids. So, I had to have a hysterectomy.

My surgeon told me that my uterus had to be "dissected out" and away from the organs, it had gummed to. The hysterectomy surgical procedure was performed successfully. After surgery, I stayed in the hospital, waiting to get well enough to go back home. I had accepted my fate and was ready to get on with my life. It was not meant to be.

Post-Hysterectomy Experience

Four days after my surgery, the doctor on ward rounds took a look at the medical charts hooked to my hospital bed's footboard and displayed a slight but perceptible frown. Yes, I caught that fleeting look.

From that point on, I had to take a series of tests. My temperature had been running high and I started to feel weak. Before the end of the day, my recovery, which appeared steady a couple of days post-surgery began to deteriorate. Blood cultures were taken and the results, which never comes soon enough, was not good.

I was immediately instructed to stop eating any food and stop drinking fluids, even before the blood culture results arrived. They took an abdominal scan and it showed images of a dark area spread around my lower digestive tract. They told me that it wasn't good, but I didn't fully understand what was going on.

I first started to feel alarmed, then I became really scared! I was immediately put on powerful antibiotics intravenously.

Then at night, the hallucinations began.

A little nap and I get horrible dreams. At night, it was never ceasing. I had bad dreams of giants, death, and deadly forms, crashing high-rises, everything trying to crush me. I dreamed of dead bodies, blood, evil, mangled giant trucks and spinning cars. Soon, I started to fear sleep and made desperate efforts to keep awake. Dreamland was utter chaos. It was literally "walking through the valley of the shadow of death".

When I complained to the doctors, they knew what was wrong. They decided to reduce my antibiotics dosage and after that, I was finally able to get some good sleep.

An Emergency Colostomy Surgery

"You've got a leak in your bowel and faecal matter is seeping into your system; septicaemia is imminent. You've got to have surgery no later than a few hours".

It was 9 pm when it became an emergency, but I still didn't understand what it was all about but from the look on my surgeon's face, I knew something was wrong. I was afraid.

The private hospital I was in lacked a well-equipped operating theatre with intensive care facilities, so arrangements were made to transfer me to the North Cross Hospital, a teaching hospital with highly equipped state-of-the-art ICU unit with professional monitoring that was next to none.

In haste, I was prepared for movement to the teaching hospital, securely strapped to a stretcher and whisked down to a waiting ambulance. That's when the realization of the danger I was in hit me. I started to feel alarmed, distressed and anxious. Was I going to die?

As the ambulance sped through the city and the paramedics ensured my comfort, we arrived at the New Cross Hospital in Wolverhampton. My brother, a paediatrician at the hospital, was there to meet us.

By 10.30 pm, pre-ops was a frenzy because it was an emergency, a matter of life and death. Needles, tubes, intravenous devices, etc..., were all fixed and attached simultaneously by about four people. I was weeping but soon felt weak. My brother was there, observing it all. I think he was allowed to stay around because he is a doctor in the same hospital.

The jabs were painful, and everything was becoming unbearable. While one nurse was trying to carefully pry off my false nails another was slapping my arm for a vein. Two pricks and I was screaming, I was in anguish. Then I hear a nurse shout, "let's leave that till she's under" and somewhere through the cobwebs of my mind, I thanked her.

By 11 pm, I was wheeled down the corridors to the operating theatre. The last thought that went through my confused mind was "Is this it, am I going to die?"

Then everything went blank!

From what I was told, the surgery lasted for about four hours and that must have been bad. When I came out from the effects of anaesthesia, I could hear faraway voices and saw fleeting images of people, but I 'wasn't there'.

Someone called my name; I think it was my surgeon. And though I still couldn't fathom what was going on, I know I heard my name.

I felt very heavy and constricted around my stomach and I could barely breathe. It felt like there were tons of bricks tied around my abdomen, or a 20kg lead weight tightly bound on my stomach. My surgeon held my hand gently and asked, "Are you okay?" I think I mumbled or nodded; I can't remember.

I was out of surgery and in ICU though I didn't know that at the time. I wasn't aware of much, neither was I aware of all the tubes, catheter, gadgets, and other such things that I was hooked to or attached to me.

A Colostomy, What's That?

I was told a colostomy procedure had been carried out, apparently as a life-saving measure, but I didn't know what a colostomy was. For the first three days in the intensive care unit, I was unaware of my colostomy, or the bag that was attached to my abdomen.

After seven days, I was taken out of the ICU and transferred to a ward with other patients who had similar ostomy problems. It was when I got to the ward that I first noticed the colostomy bag stuck to my abdomen.

Then I met a young colostomy patient who spoke to me and told me about her colostomy. I was still in a daze. There was also my Stoma nurse who carefully explained what my condition was all about, what the bag attached to my abdomen was, how to wear it, and how it worked.

That was when I burst into tears, finally understanding the procedure I just had and why I had to wear a shit bag.

I Was in Denial

My Stoma Nurse removed the colostomy bag and I saw my stoma for the first time. I nearly puked at the raw cherry-like button that was the outlet through which my faeces will be expelled. I took my eyes away from it, but the nurse fully understood my reaction. That was when she introduced me to the young lady, about half my age, who was on admission for a colostomy reversal.

The young lady spoke to me about her own experience and how she lived with it. She promised me that I'll think nothing of it after a few weeks and told me how nobody needs ever know I have a colostomy, except, of course, those I want to tell.

She told me how she still went to parties, wore her jeans, and generally do all the things her age group does. She said she continued to live her life as she did before her colostomy surgery.

Certainly, she was an inspiration. She successfully encouraged me and made begin to accept my condition.

Some Good News - My Colostomy was Reversible

My surgeon had told me my colostomy was reversible, but he also told me I'd have to wait at least a year before an ostomy reconnect.

Because my body had gone through so much trauma, undergoing two major operations within a week, my body needed to heal completely. Plus, I still had the hysterectomy wounds, a deep cut running from my midriff down to my lower abdomen.

Plus, I was opened up in the same cut line for the colostomy procedure just a few days after my hysterectomy surgery. However, this time around, the cut area was not sutured back, but tacked together in a few spots and allowed to heal naturally. Did it look gory? Yes, it did.

My doctor told me that he tries not to perform a colostomy reversal in less than 12 months to give the body ample time to heal completely. He said that within a year, my colon will have healed completely and by then, I'll be ready and strong enough to withstand another major surgery. It made so much sense.

Physical and Emotional Recovery

My physical and emotional recovery was slow. It was a big challenge, learning how to use a colostomy bag and the other colostomy supplies. Over a week after moving into the ward, I was still not allowed any food because the stoma hadn't started to function. Peristalsis must be confirmed through auscultation (listening to sounds with a stethoscope) for intestinal movements before food consumption is allowed.

I was hungry and longed for food consumed through my mouth but instead, I was 'fed' a thick whitish fluid intravenously, through a tube fixed into an artery at the base of my neck. It is a delicate procedure that is highly prone to infection, but all went well with that aspect of my feeding. The only problem was I had to have it on for many hours, making moving around very clumsy.

Meanwhile, I was put on painkillers that were self-regulated. All I had to do was press a button to release the painkillers into my body whenever the pain increased or became unbearable.

Then one day I felt 'wind' passing out through the stoma into the colostomy bag. It sounded like indescribable sounds that come out from a baby's mouth. My Stoma nurse seemed pleased and expected me to be as well. "The organ is working," she told me. This was the second hurdle to cross, the first being surgery itself.

Was I pleased? I'm not sure I was at the time. The good part, however, was that I was put back on solid foods and could eat orally. I was given jelly and light broths to start with and they tasted 'heavenly', after being starved for many days. Now I'll have to start putting into practice what I've been taught by my Stoma Nurse.

For the first couple of days after the first wind was expelled, there was nothing. It became a waiting game but eventually, the awaited human waste started to seep out.

My stoma bag was changed and a new one fitted a few days after my first excrement after surgery. The nurses had to help because, at my first attempt, I burst into tears. It was like there was no way I could handle this, and I didn't feel like trying either.

Eventually, I did try to change my bag myself, and soon enough, I became adept at it that I amazed the nurses. Before I left the hospital, after being on admission for about four weeks, I became confident about managing my colostomy, could change my bag in minutes, and had learned what it entails to care for my stoma.

7 Reasons Why You May Need a Colostomy Surgical Procedure

Before I delve further, let me just explain some of the reasons why you may need a colostomy surgical procedure. The colostomy procedure is performed as a life-saving measure that may be linked to various illnesses or conditions. In this procedure, a section of the colon is diverted and then attached to a stoma, which is a hole made in the abdominal wall. This opening, the colostomy stoma, enables a patient to expel faeces from the digestive tract because the bowels and rectum have been surgically disabled.

There are many reasons why a patient may need to undergo colostomy surgery but the seven most common reasons why anyone may require this surgical procedure is if they have:

1. Diverticulitis
2. Crohn's disease

3. Cancer of the bowels
4. Obstruction of the bowels
5. Trauma and/or injury
6. An emergency
7. Bowel incontinence

1. Diverticulitis

In diverticulitis, the diverticula, small pouches in the walls of the colon, get inflamed and then infected. The onset of this will give symptoms such as:

- Severe pain in the stomach
- Extremely high temperature
- Vomiting

With severe or repeated diverticulitis disease, a patient's doctor may feel there is a need to remove the affected section of the colon and reattached the remaining part of it. And because the colon will heal naturally, but needs some time, a patient may require a colostomy stoma as a temporary measure.

2. Crohn's Disease

Crohn's disease is a condition that causes inflammation of the digestive tract. Symptoms include:

- Abdominal pain
- Diarrhoea

Patients with cases of Crohn's disease can be treated without surgery, but if there is no response to treatment, colon surgery will have to be performed, by surgically removing a section of the bowel and performing a temporary colostomy procedure.

3. Cancer of the Bowels

Cancer of the bowels is one of the most common cancers in the developed world, with thousands of new cases occurring each year. They mostly develop within the rectum or the colon, and this condition is referred to as colorectal cancer. Colostomy surgery is the most common form of treatment, where the affected portion of the bowel is surgically removed. With the removal of the diseased part, the remaining colon is then reattached, and a temporary colostomy stoma 'installed' to perform waste (faeces) elimination duties.

The temporary ostomy will be in use for times ranging from four months to a couple of years, depending on the physician's recommendations, and the patient's condition. With reversible colostomy surgery, the colostomy and stoma will be removed, and the healed colon is reactivated.

However, with colorectal cancer, if the problem is within the rectum, and it has to be removed, the patient will likely require a permanent colostomy. This form of colostomy procedure is irreversible.

4. Obstruction of the Bowels

An obstruction in the bowel is a serious condition and must be treated as a medical emergency. This is because there is the risk of bowel rupture, which in turn will cause a serious infection and many times, internal bleeding. The ways that the passageway of the bowel can become blocked include:

- Acute constipation
- Bowel cancer
- Scarring of the bowel the lining (due to infection or inflammation)
- Hernia

With severe bowel obstruction or rupture, it may become necessary to remove either a portion of the colon, in which case, a temporary colostomy will be performed. However, if all of the colon is removed, the patient will require a permanent colostomy surgery.

5. Trauma and Injury

Experience of severe damage by a penetrating injury to the colon, for example, a gunshot wound, a knife stab, or a gruesome accident to the abdominal area, may require the colon to be removed. Depending on the degree of injury, a temporary or permanent colostomy surgical procedure may be performed.

6. An Emergency Situation

Some patients, in hospital for surgery related to other conditions, may wake up to discover they have a colostomy stoma. This most likely occurred during that involves dissection close to the colon (in my experience, for example, I was a female patient with massive fibroids who came to the hospital to have them removed).

Larger and numerous fibroid tissues may have encouraged the entire uterus 'gumming' to nearby organs. And in trying to remove these fibroids, the colon may have been cut (accidentally) or nicked. If after surgery, there is an indication of severe infection, there is the likelihood of seepage of faeces into the body system. With this, a temporary colostomy may have to be done to save the patient's life. The colostomy reversal may then be carried out after some months.

7. Bowel Incontinence

Bowel incontinence is a medical condition whereby patients are unable to control their bowel movement, thereby experiencing episodes of embarrassing soiling. This condition is more common with the elderly. A colostomy surgery may be used as a 'last resort' medical measure if all other medical or surgical procedures prove unsuccessful.

What to Expect After the Procedure?

As it was in my case, after surgery, you'll feel heavy and tight around your abdomen and you'll also feel a lot of pain and feel extremely weak. You will be on intravenous pain relievers that will help the pain reduce to the barest minimum. You will soon be aware of the colostomy bag attached to your abdomen and depending on your physical and mental condition; your doctor will carefully explain your current condition and tell you what to expect.

For the first few days, you won't be able to stand on your own two feet and it's virtually impossible to take a shower. You will be towel-washed by the nurses and you will have to contend with some discomfort.

At first, your stoma will not function and because you haven't started to eat solid foods, you won't pass out waste through the newly installed stoma. As a post-surgery patient, you will not be allowed to eat or drink anything until the stoma starts to function.

When your stoma starts to function varies from one patient to another but in my case, it took about a week. Peristalsis (involuntary constriction and relaxation of the muscles of the intestine) must be confirmed through auscultation (listening to sounds with a stethoscope) of the patient's stomach for intestinal movements. As soon as the intestinal movement is ascertained, you can start to 'eat' your first meal which will be clear liquids. It soon progresses to eating softer foods like broths.

A couple of days after colostomy surgery, once conditions are favourable, you will be encouraged to sit up in bed though you will have to be lifted (you can't do this simple task on your own) to achieve this. Depending on your strength and willpower, you will be encouraged to try standing up unaided. Soon enough, you should be able to take a few steps, aided by a nurse.

It is particularly important to start this early process as it encourages early healing and a faster recovery.

Coping with My Emotional State after Colostomy Surgery

How do you cope with your emotions after colostomy surgery and how do you come to terms with living with a stoma? At first, it is hard to come to terms with having a s**t bag stuck to your abdomen; what can be worse than that? Going through emotional stress is expected, but how do you deal with it?

After surgery, your emotions are probably all over the place; it will be a difficult time for you. You may feel a sense of hopelessness at this seemingly horrendous situation and the emotional stress will be compounded with the realization of having to live a life, temporarily or permanently without having control over defecating. This is exactly how I felt for the first couple of weeks. Dejected, sad, and weepy. These feelings are normal and should be expected.

Depending on age, occupation, lifestyle, profession, and a few other factors, ostomates will react to the condition in different ways, but generally, the thoughts that go through our minds are fundamentally the same. You are not alone!

How it Affects Us Emotionally

Some ostomates keep their feelings to themselves and appear withdrawn from everyone and everything that used to be of interest to them, but others are quite open-minded about their condition. They have no reservations about expressing their feelings and concerns with members of their family and friends.

It is important that you first try to accept the fact as soon as is possible and the earlier you come to terms with having to live with a stoma, whether temporarily or permanently, the better it is for your state of mind.

It is important that you avoid feeling or doing these following things:

1. Feeling like the whole world knows your condition.

2. Withdraw into yourself.
3. Bottle up your emotions.
4. Become self-conscious.
5. Become anti-social.
6. Change your lifestyle.
7. Feel a sense of shame.
8. Worry about what people say.
9. Stop your recreational activities.
10. Change your fashion style.

Help and Support for Ostomates

Yes, courage takes guts, but the good thing to know is that no colostomy patient has to deal with this alone.

Group support is always available from Stoma (Ostomy) Associations in your region. If you are a colostomy patient or a carer for ostomates, if you need a list of contacts, ask your Stoma Nurse, or seek additional information online.

If you have worries, fears, questions, or just a shoulder to lean on once in a while, get your thought out into the open. You can talk to your Stoma Nurse, fellow ostomates online, or join an ostomy patients' forums. Talking about your colostomy and discussing it with like minds will help assuage your negative feelings and calm your mind.

With time, once you've mastered how to manage your stoma, you will be more relaxed about it. And even if you still feel uncomfortable to be around people, fearing they'll know, you will eventually find that you've got nothing to worry about. People never notice. Once you recognise the few common problems that may occur and learn how to avoid or reduce them to the barest minimum, you'll be more than fine.

Online communities are the best places to be and interact if you are emotionally affected by having to live with a stoma. It's only on such forums that you get to share thoughts and experiences with fellow ostomates. This form of interaction will enlighten you to the fact that you are not the only one going through this emotional crisis.

The Importance of Making Emotional Progress

As an ostomy patient, not making emotional progress will affect your quality of life negatively, and you don't want that. If you feel helpless, seek advice from the professionals (doctor or stoma nurse) or join an ostomy support group. Information on finding and getting advice can be provided by your Stoma Care Nurse who most probably will be the first person to point out these issues.

Most likely, there will also be care and understanding from family and friends that know about your condition. However, the most important thing is to be positive about your stoma. Have a sense of realism; it will go a long way in helping you manage your condition and accept stoma care as a part of your routine and lifestyle.

Having a stoma is not a hindrance in any way whatsoever, and it, therefore, should not be seen as an obstacle in either your personal or professional life. Just learn to be resilient.

Don't Be a Slave to Your Feelings

Within the first few weeks of your surgical procedure, you should have accepted your condition. Okay, maybe this is easier said than done and varies from one patient to the other, but it is true, you will, eventually. You may still be in the process of learning how to effectively manage a stoma, and how to recognize the workings of your digestive system, depending on your type of diet, but then that's normal.

One thing about a stoma is that you'll never have that feeling of 'wanting to go'. The stoma seems to have a mind of its own and empties your waste as, and when it pleases and that can be worrying. But you will soon get accustomed to it.

And though managing your ostomy will be confusing at first, and you will have many questions and issues arising like:

- What's the fastest way to empty or change a colostomy bag without making a mess?
- Can I travel without worrying about unpleasant incidences?
- How do I prevent bag ballooning?
- How will I manage gas build-up in my colostomy bag?
- How do I guard against leaks?
- Will I be able to swim with a stoma?

Some of these issues are elaborated upon, further down in this book.

Dealing with such physical issues will become easier once you have come to terms with the condition. Coping with the condition demands patience and the determination to look on the bright side of things. Remember, it could be worse. You may have died in the operating room but now, you are lucky to have the chance of living a good life.

Think about this. If you weren't fortunate enough to have good medical care, what would have happened and without your colostomy surgery, what would have been your chances of survival? Perhaps, very slim.

My Colostomy Food and Diet Tips

If you have an ostomy, you probably want to know if you have to make major changes to your regular diet, or not. As an ex-colostomy patient, I can only tell you of my experience and the nutritional pattern I followed. So, if you've just had a colostomy and wonder if you can still enjoy your favourite foods and drinks, I can say yes and no.

Yes, because there are a few simple nutritional rules that you can follow that will make the digestion of what you consume, and its elimination as waste, easy on your stoma and general condition.

No, because, with a colostomy, there doesn't have to be a change in your regular diet, perhaps what you will need to is to modify it.

What it boils down to is that it is more about what to expect when you eat certain foods, as opposed to whether a certain food is good for your condition, or not. It doesn't matter whether you had a permanent or reversible procedure; what you can eat in the two instances remains the same.

Before your discharge from the hospital, your Stoma Nurse will have instructed you on how to use ostomy supplies that will now become a part of your everyday life and there would have been mention of your nutritional diet and how best to balance it.

As an ostomate, whatever you drink or eat must be tolerable to your digestive system, especially in the first few weeks after surgery but after that initial period, you can eat whatever you've been eating pre-surgery, but you may have to take certain foods and drinks in moderation.

Foods for colostomy patients must be balanced, just as it should have been before your operation. For instance, if you were a junk foodie in the past, you will have to reduce its consumption drastically; same as it applies to people without a condition.

However, as in everyday life, every individual has his or her favourite foods and this applies to stoma patients as well.

This is not to say that there won't be a few that demand a special nutritional plan. The reason for surgery in the first place, must be considered and a special diet may be necessary because of this, and not just because you had a colostomy. In such cases, diet plans can be individualised and will depend on other factors, including other health challenges if any, weight, lifestyle, and age.

Having said that, the important recommendations I can give you in terms of diet, nutrition, and eating habits are quite simple to follow:

Consumption

Consume smaller meal portions every day. Eating four to six smaller meals a day is much more beneficial in that it allows for improved absorption of the necessary nutrients in the foods, and it also ensures that the elimination of waste is easy and effortless.

Fibre intake

Reduce your fibre intake. Wheat products like oats, maize, and wholegrain breakfast cereals, all high in fibre, must be taken in moderation. Eliminating waste resulting from the consumption of excessive fibre is hard on the stoma, especially in the early weeks following surgery. The hard stool will be too stressful on a recovering bowel. It is best to wait until your Stoma Nurse or the doctor says it is okay to consume fibrous foods and vegetables. In my case, I was of such foods for the first six weeks.

Mastication

Chew your food thoroughly and completely, whether it is tender meat, chicken, fish, raw carrots, nuts, etc... Mastication must be complete. You don't want your stoma "popping" out corn kernels! Thorough chewing is the most important aspect of a post colostomy surgery diet. It has been said that the recommended number of times that food must be chewed before swallowing is not less than 25 times. And this especially applies to beef. Proper mouth-grinding of food allows for better absorption and easy digestion, making waste elimination easy on the stoma.

J Pouch diet

This ostomy diet which consists of soft foods are great and gentle on the stomach. They include highly nutritional smoothies, blended juices, thick soups, broths with chunks of vegetables, and slowly cooked menus. These digest faster, easier, and better and makes waste elimination virtually stress-free for your stoma.

What to avoid

If you can, try to avoid fruits, drinks, or foods with high acidic content. If on the other hand, you cannot, take them in moderation or keep its consumption to the barest minimum. However, moderation is key.

Fluids

To avoid the risk of dehydration, take a minimum of seven glasses of water a day. If you love fruit juices, you can substitute a couple of glasses of water with non-acidic fruit juices. The colon absorbs water in the body and when it is undergoing a healing process, though it may not be functional because of your colostomy, additional water intake is essential.

Beef and poultry

Meat, chicken, and other animal products must be cooked tender. Cut them into small pieces before popping them into your mouth because larger tougher pieces may clog the stoma. Some colostomy patients have had to return to the hospital for complications arising from an obstructed stoma and you don't want that to happen to you.

Food and Drinks Guide

STOMA OBSTRUCTIVE	ODOUR PRODUCING	INCREASED/LOOSE STOOL	GAS PRODUCING
Apple peels	Asparagus	Alcoholic beverages	Alcoholic beverages
Raw cabbage	Baked beans	Whole grains	Carbonated drinks
Celery	Broccoli	Bran cereals	Beans
Chinese vegetables	Cabbage	Cooked cabbage	Soy
Whole kernels corn	Cod liver oil	Fresh fruits	Cabbage
Coconuts	Eggs	Leafy greens	Cauliflower
Dried fruits	Fish	Milk	Cucumbers
Mushrooms	Garlic	Prunes	Dairy products
Oranges	Onions	Raisins	Chewing gum
Nuts	Peanut butter	Raw vegetables	Milk
Pineapples	Some vitamins	Spices	Nuts
Popcorn	Strong cheese	Apple and prune juice	Onions
CONSTIPATION RELIEF	**ODOUR CONTROL**	**LOOSE STOOL CONTROL**	**FLATULENCE REDUCING**
Coffee	Buttermilk	Apple sauce	Fennel tea
Cooked fruits	Cranberry juice	Very ripe bananas	Cranberry juice
Cooked vegetables	Orange juice	Boiled rice	Buttermilk
Fresh juices	Parsley	Peanut butter	Peppermint oil
Fresh fruits	Tomato juice	Tapioca	
Water	Yoghurt	Toast	**STOOL COLOUR CHANGES**
Mild laxative	Peppermint oil	White bread	
		Potatoes	Asparagus
		Crackers	Beet
		Pasta	Food colouring
		Weak tea	Iron capsules
		Marshmallows	Liquorice
		Jelly babies	Strawberries
			Tomato sauce

If you wish, draw up a menu on a pin-up board and stick with it. It will help you to keep track of what you eat. You can also check the colostomy nutritional guide above for help in planning what to eat, how much of it is good for you, and how each type of food works and reacts in your body.

You should detect your pattern a few weeks after surgery and know what may be good or bad for your stoma. By that time, you will have had a good idea of the timing of your bowel movements as well. From my experience, I found that food or drink intake triggers off my stoma and waste starts to spew into my colostomy bag.

A colostomy diet plan must, however, be seen only as a guide that will help you manage and cope with the challenges of living with a stoma. Following these simple rules will ensure that you'll be fine.

J Pouch Diet

When the colon and rectum are surgically removed, a pouch or reservoir must be created for the excretion of stool; its exit from the body. This surgically created reservoir in the shape of the letter 'J', is an option for selected patients.

The term 'J Pouch diet' is another name used to describe a colostomy diet and is highly recommended and approved by the UOAA (United Ostomy Associations of America), a member of the International Ostomy Association and a national organisation that makes provision for information, support, and advocacy for colostomy patients and their carer.

Useful Tips

- Eat and drink moderately.
- There are no special foods to eat or not.
- It's more about the types of foods and drinks to avoid or take in moderation.
- Carbonated drinks will cause colostomy bag ballooning, a gas build-up.
- Be content with just half a glass of fizzy drinks.
- Eat steak sparingly. It can cause constipation which puts a strain on your stoma.
- Eating healthy will help patients of a temporary colostomy heal faster.

How I Coped with Wearing Bags and Managing a Stoma

How does one cope with wearing colostomy bags? If you asked me a week after my procedure, I'll tell you I wish I were dead! But then, a few weeks down the line and I soon became an expert at managing a stoma. It's not so bad after all. This means that it did not take me that long to learn how to cope with wearing colostomy bags. I remember when I first walked out through the hospital doors that cold winter evening after spending weeks there and undergoing two major operations. On my way out, I think I felt a little more confident about managing my stoma.

The initial after-surgery shock soon wore off and with acceptance and adaption to my new condition, I had decided to quickly get over it and learn to live with a colostomy. After that long four-week stay, I had learned how to wear, take care of, and fix, drain or change colostomy bags.

But when I got back home, I lost some of that confidence I had built up. There were no nurses around to help, pamper, and take care of me. There were no more confidence-building pep talks about how easy it is to live with and manage a colostomy.

The First Few Weeks at Home

I had expected the emotional stress because I had been prepared for what to expect and apparently, this feeling is a normal post-surgery mood. All I thought about was my stoma and how my lifestyle may be altered because of my colostomy. It took a few weeks to adapt to the life of living with a stoma and with the benefit of hindsight; it truly was a passing phase.

I found myself learning more about my condition by doing extensive research on how life is like living with a colostomy. And as I discovered better and more efficient ways to manage by myself, I knew I was now in full control and able to tackle any unexpected situation. But then, there were quite a few unanticipated circumstances now and then which ranged from colostomy bag ballooning, caused by the consumption of certain diets to pancaking and bag-blowouts.

Eating and General Diet

I barely ate any food, hoping that eating much less will ensure the stoma bag is filled with as little waste as is possible, but that wasn't so wise because I had to eat well. I was just out of the hospital and needed to build up my body mass, strength, and stamina plus I needed to put on some weight. I had lost about 10 kilos.

I bought a food blender and ate mostly blended foods for breakfast and dinner which consisted of fruits, vegetables, and nut mixes. But I soon stuck to a simple diet eating most foods I love but in moderation. I was bent on ensuring that waste was expelled with ease and at a reduced amount.

Clothing

I had to modify the way I dressed and that certainly bothered me a lot. I stored away my tight-fitting clothes (a body-con outfit fan) and opted for looser fitting apparel, especially those that are a bit loose around the waist.

Trousers, shorts, and casual pants posed a problem initially, but I soon found that low-rise pants worked better for me as it allowed my colostomy bag to hang out unhindered by waistbands.

I love Palazzo pants, and these were my favourites for that first couple of weeks. They were loose and free and looked good on too. I brought out my loose tops and also bought some new fashionable loosely fitting blouses, designer T-shirts which I sometimes tied into a knot at one side and bust fitting but flared short jackets.

I also invested in long scarves and chic fashionable wraps. I'd drape them over one shoulder and casually throw it over the other in that chic lady-like way, all to conceal my colostomy bag if it balloons. Shirt dresses and shifts worked beautifully and concealed the fact that you have a stoma bag on.

Sleep

I couldn't sleep soundly the first few days because there was the horrible thought that lying on my stomach might burst my bag and splatter its contents all over my sheets. I had to learn to sleep on my side and I eventually inculcated that way of sleeping within a few days of my arrival at home.

At the hospital, it was a different 'kettle of fish'. There were always nurses around to help you out of nasty situations that may occur.

When you are in bed with your partner, the last thing you wish to happen is a burst or leaking bag whilst being fast asleep.

Partying and Socialising

My first outing was funny enough dinner at a restaurant, and this was just a couple of weeks out of the hospital. The food looked really good, but I barely ate for the fear of those 'farty gas' sounds that always came on unexpectedly. I feared my colostomy bag may fill up rapidly (this always happens after a meal), I may have some leakage. It wasn't an easy outing at the time and though I was all smiles and cheery, 99% of the guests never knew a thing about my condition.

My next outing was a party, and I mean a disco party where we practically danced all night long. I was a bit apprehensive about attending, but I'm quite brave and strong enough to face major challenges, so, I decided to face this one too.

I was dressed to-the-hilt and had a wonderful time. For a few hours, I forgot all about my stoma and colostomy bag, but I had 'armed' myself with two extra bags in case I had to have a change sometime through the night. I never needed to use them.

Travelling

I had to travel by air six weeks after I left the hospital and I wasn't looking forward to that. It was a six-hour flight and I was going from a very cold climate into a very hot and humid one.

From the time I left home to the time I got to my destination, I'd be spending ten hours in airports and in the air. That thought made me panic briefly, but it had no choice.

I had more than enough colostomy supplies in my hand luggage, including a small can of deodorant, wipes, and ten colostomy bags (yes, 10!), all neatly packed in a zippered designer colostomy supplies bag. I had to pre-cut the holes on the bag's face-plate because scissors were not allowed in any hand luggage.

Any ostomy patient will know what it's like changing a colostomy pouch in any public toilet. The odour spreads the second you pull off the faceplate. But changing or emptying a pouch in an aeroplane's toilet is something else entirely. The odour was so consuming, and the deodorants couldn't hide the smell. I was like, "Oh well, it's just too bad". I had to change three times before I got to my destination.

One thing was for sure though; I was getting more adept at this and spent less time than I would have if I had to use a toilet the normal way.

Major Challenges I Faced Wearing Colostomy Bags

The first few days at home. Wearing, changing, and managing was a great challenge and it took some getting used to. Eventually, 'we' all got along fine together, colostomy bags, my stoma, and I. However, there were issues that I encountered, and these issues were accompanied by some worries.

1. Knowing the right time to change a colostomy pouch.
2. Dealing with the stench every time a bag needs a change or a drain (ostomy deodorants never worked well for me).
3. Worrying about colostomy bag ballooning or leaks.
4. Wondering if a blowout is imminent!
5. Worrying about running out of supplies. It is a major disaster if you run out of stoma bags.
6. Bleeding around the stoma outer ring.

7. Loud embarrassing sounds of gas emanating from the stoma into the bag. I call it farting-into-the-bag.
8. How to dispose of used ostomy bags. Because of this, I preferred to wear the drainable systems.
9. The horrible feeling of self-consciousness that never seems to go away.

The first week I was 'in and out' of the bathroom, checking, sniffing, worrying about the fluid scanty stool. I soon discovered that bags I can drain worked best for me. The ease of draining loose stool from pouches through the drainage opening was super.

The Velcro tape tabs were always strong and secure, contrary to my initial thoughts that they may pop open and unravel. Gladly, this never happened because the ends are folded over a couple of times before being secured with the Velcro tape.

Back to My Regular Lifestyle with my Colostomy

After fully accepting my condition mentally, I must say that I found that it beats having to use the toilet the normal way. There were a few times when the urge to go the normal way occurred and at first it was alarming. After talking to my doctor, I was assured that it was normal. Because of the accumulation of mucus in the rectum despite its being idle, the urge to expel something occurs occasionally.

My doctor advised I try to expel the mucus build-up by sitting on the toilet and bearing down lightly and that if something doesn't pop out, I should use a very mild suppository that will aid its expulsion.

In no time, managing my colostomy became second nature. It gave me a new lease on life. I had come to terms with having a stoma, and my initial reaction and shock after my surgery had been replaced by happier thoughts.

All this while, only a couple of people knew I was walking around with a colostomy bag on. And because I watched what I ate and kept to a simple diet, I hardly experienced constipation, leaks, or blowouts. In the space of twelve months, I only experienced blowouts about three times.

Ballooning was still a common occurrence and usually happened whenever I consume fizzy or alcoholic drinks like sodas, sparkling wines, or champagne. When this gas build-up occurs, I just sneak into the toilet and let out the gas through the end drain of the drainable colostomy bag and I'm all done in two minutes!

Living with a colostomy wasn't so bad after all. After the initial three months, I was beginning to enjoy my colostomy bag. I used modern colostomy bags in skin colour, and they looked so cute and neat.

With only 9 months to go before my reverse colostomy, I was as happy as can be. And because my husband was my pillar of support, adjusting was easy. When he first saw my colostomy bag pouch attached to my abdomen, guess what he said - "it looks so sexy". I didn't think so then, but who was I to argue?

How I Kept My Stoma Clean, to Avoid Infection

As an ostomate, caring for your stoma and ensuring that it is clean and germ-free is an important part of a stoma care routine. A clean stoma will guard against bacteria that may result in irritation, or worse, an infection. Learn how to keep your stoma hygienic and infection-free.

After an ostomy procedure and your discharge from the hospital, taking care of your stoma is a routine you'll need to master because the nurses are no more there to give you a helping hand.

While I was in the hospital, my Stoma Nurse was always there to walk me through every detail of stoma care and management and with her kind and encouraging words, I was able to gain more confidence in myself and come to terms with my condition.

But every colostomy patient is different. While some will build up their confidence enough to easily take off from where the nurses left, it's not that easy for others.

The days that follow your colostomy procedure can be confusing and challenging and there seems to be so much to learn but one of the most important lessons you'll need to know is how to take proper care of the stoma.

How to Clean a Stoma

The stoma acts as an opening through which human waste in the form of faeces or urine is expelled and so, it requires constant but gentle cleaning. From experience, I found that cleaning my stoma every time I changed my colostomy bag helped me avoid infections and through the duration of my temporary colostomy, my stoma was never infected, even when I had bruising.

Because waste passes through this opening, you must try to guard against is bruising. It is easy to accidentally bruise your stoma through scratching around its perimeter, pinching it, scrubbing too hard with a sponge, or from face-plate holes that are cut too tight.

Though it may look raw, moist, and sensitive, a stoma has no sensory nerves. This means it is devoid of nerve endings and therefore insensitive to touch, pain, or excessively hot water.

Most of the time, the bleeding is usually slight and will stop. However, if you do have bad bruising that leads to bleeding, contact your doctor. That's what I did. With my condition, he told me I had no reason to get alarmed as long as I keep it clean. Cleaning around the stoma is not hard and the following ways will show you the methods I employed to keep my stoma clean and germs free:

1. Wash your hands before cleaning your stoma.
2. Gently clean the stoma with the wipes that come with your ostomy supplies.
3. Clean the folds and crevices where bits of faeces or stale urine may be stuck.
4. Clean the skin around the stoma. This is the pancake area where a colostomy bag's faceplate is attached.
5. Use a fresh sheet of wipes for every step.
6. If you experience any faecal leakage on your skin, wipe it off and clean thoroughly with dampened wipes.
7. You can shower without your ostomy bag if you wish and give your stoma a gentle wash. However, expect some waste to be expelled while showering.

8. Use lukewarm water in the absence of wipes. Because the stoma has no pain sensors, don't use hot water, to avoid scalding.
9. Carry out this stoma care routine a minimum of two times a day.
10. Wash your hands after your stoma care process.

If you are a mother caring for a young child with an ostomy, or a caregiver taking care of an elderly person with challenges, the patient's Stoma Nurse will instruct you on everything you need to know, like how to care for a stoma, how to use appliances, how to deal with/watch out for ostomy-associated mishaps, and how to be encouraging to the patient by lifting their spirits.

Supplies Required to Keep a Stoma Clean

Wipes

You will always need a lot of wipes because every time you change your stoma bag, you will need wipes to clean around the stoma. When leaks occur, you also need wipes. Before you use your wipes, ensure you dampen it with clean warm water before using it to clean the stoma and its surrounds. There are pre-moistened wipes that you can use but they may contain products that will irritate your skin. It is a great idea to stick to dry wipes that can serve as washcloths. They should NOT be re-used after each use. Avoid using paper towels or tissues to clean the stoma. These will leave little bits of paper stuck in the moist folds or crevices of the stoma.

Mild soap

Mild, non-perfumed soap is best to cleanse the stoma and the surrounding areas if it is visibly soiled, or if bits of faeces is caked around the perimeter. It is best to purchase your soap with your regular ostomy supplies. Don't use just bath soap of other soaps as it may irritate the area. If you have to, check the ingredients in the soap before use. Avoid harsh skin cleansers that have alcohol because alcohol will irritate your stoma and the skin around it. If you have to pancake, one of the colostomy problems that happen often, clean the area with mild soap.

Shower protector

If you prefer to shower with your pouch off, it's good to consider using a stoma shower protector after you may have cleaned the stoma with clear water.

This will protect your stoma from perfumed shower gels or bubble bath soaps if you decide to have a long soak. Additionally, this protector will keep waste from leaking into your bathwater.

Deodorant

You want to have a canister of deodorant while cleaning your stoma. What I did was spray a couple of spurts around my abdomen before removing my colostomy bag, then another few bursts while cleaning my stoma opening to empty or changing. After, I spray some around the bathroom to take care of lingering odour, especially if it's a public toilet in a mall or a restaurant.

Tips

- If you cut your faceplate holes, remember that the hole is meant to fit fairly snug around the stoma. Many ostomates cut this opening too small and this will squeeze the stoma tightly which in turn will cause bruising and slight bleeding. This may trigger off an infection.
- If the hole is wider than the stoma, the surrounding skin will become exposed to clumps of human waste. This will cause irritation and/or become infected.
- Excessive changing, pulling, tugging or yanking the faceplate off the skin will pull at abdominal hairs. The constant pull and tug will cause skin irritation for some, so, if you have a hairy abdomen, shave the area occasionally.

Having read all this, you will find that caring for your stoma is a necessary but easy task. Once you start to get the hang of it, you can care for your stoma and manage it successfully.

Problems to Expect as an Ostomate

As a colostomy patient, you will experience a few challenging situations that are best described as minor mishaps. What are they, when do they occur, and how can you overcome them or keep them to the barest minimum? Find out in this article.

If you have a colostomy, there are some challenging situations you must expect. Some of them are quite funny, some embarrassing, and a few, disastrous. Even though this may appear worrisome, they are not serious issues and therefore not worth worrying about. Here, you will find the major problems to expect, how to manage them, and how to overcome them. Being an ex-ostomate myself, who has been there, I can tell you about the situations I had to face and conquer, and the ones that gave me some concern, and also let you know how I managed and eventually overcame them.

- Flatulence
- Loose stool
- Colostomy bag leaks
- Discomfort in the rectum
- Faceplate absorbing water
- Pancaking
- Bag 'blowouts'

Flatulence

This is a funny one. I found that passing gas into my colostomy bag was a comic relief of sorts. Why do I say this? Because gas passing out through the stoma is hardly ever silent. It can be acutely noisy. For some strange reason, it always reminded me of a burbling baby, something that sounds like blowing bubbles, quite cute but noisy.

Before the gas is expelled, you will get a funny feeling in your tummy, a 10 to 15-second warning to let you know it's on its way, then finally erupting into your bag. Learn to recognize this pre-farting feeling.

The not-so-funny side is that the sound IS loud enough to attract anyone within earshot, or someone sitting on the sofa across from you, but to handle this problem, I just had to approach it with some sense of humour.

How did I overcome this? If I am within earshot, which as usual, I simply chuckle or start to speak when the warning signs approach. I'll say something like "sorry about this. I recently had a surgical procedure and I don't have much control over this bubbling sound for now". Surprisingly no-one visitor or stranger has ever asked about the sound, and if they did wonder, I will never know which was good enough for me.

A good tip is to lay off the fizzy drinks. They are an absolute disaster if you take some when you go visiting, to a party, or go out with friends.

Loose/Watery Stool

You will soon discover that foods with high levels of roughage like some fruits, cereals, and salads, for instance, are among the most efficient foods and produce the least amount of stool by ostomates. If you have to go out, these are good foods to eat before venturing out anywhere, or to a function. With these type of foods, your bag won't fill up unexpectedly and you won't need to go back and forth to the toilet for a change, a bag drain.

On the other hand, junk food like fast foods, rich restaurant dishes, beans, and such tend to produce the most waste, concerning consumption. So, watch what you eat before you go on an outing, to school, or work.

Try to study your system to know which foods take longer to process in your digestive system, and which ones don't. What I did was to keep a mental note of my observations and adhere strictly to the kind of *colostomy diet* and made it a routine.

At the time, a fellow ostomy patient told me this, "you don't want to eat pork and beans five hours before you go to a quiet church service, neither would you want to eat a fast-food lunch if you were planning to travel on a long road trip". The loose stool will fill your colostomy bag in no time, so, plan your meals according to your daily lined up activities especially if you an individual who is always on-the-move. This way, you will avoid embarrassing situations, and you will be able to keep your inconveniences to the barest minimum.

Bag Leaks

This one is nasty and is one mishap you don't want to encounter, especially when you are outdoors. When bag leaks happen, faeces seep out through an open bubble in the colostomy bag's faceplate, and the very first thing you will notice is a slight whiff of faecal matter. You won't miss that tell-tale odour, no way will it go by unnoticed.

Immediately you smell something, go and change your bag and replace the waxy faceplate if you are using a two-piece appliance. Never, ever dismiss this because it will gradually, within seconds, get worse and the odour will spread before you know it. To avoid the embarrassment, use a seal ring. With a seal ring fitted, you can be doubly sure there' will be no leakages and no seeping odour. With seal rings, you can take a long bubble bath without worrying about a swelling faceplate causing leaking of gas or faeces.

I barely had any bag-leak problem and because I can detect smell faster than a bloodhound, I'm up and off to the loo before anyone notices. When I am far away from a public or private toilet, which is unusual, I know I'm in deep you-know-what, and so will you, so, take extra care to ensure your bag's face-plate is firmly secured. If you are lucky, you won't be in that situation often. I was fortunate not to be.

Ensure you carry along with you at least two spare colostomy bags and one faceplate (if you use the two-piece appliance) AT ALL TIMES. I usually had double that number with me. You can never be too careful. If a leak or blowout occurs, having enough spares will be a real lifesaver.

Discomfort in the Rectum

I vividly remember the first time I had discomfort in my rectum. It was a weird feeling of wanting to go to the toilet to defecate and it was least expected because that area is supposed to have been sealed shut in my abdomen. It was so alarming that I had to call my doctor.

He calmed me down and told me that such was expected with some colostomy patients, but it is not a common occurrence. It can happen to some ostomates and not happen with others. He claimed that once in a while, I may eliminate rectally when I get this feeling. He recommended I use a very mild suppository and I did.

That is how I learned that the rectum will still produce mucus and when it accumulates, you'll feel the I-need-to-go feeling. It has to be eliminated when it accumulates but the good thing is that if it happens at all, it only happens once in a while for most ostomates and what finally pops out is hardly larger than a grape.

If you experience this, don't panic; it is normal. If it doesn't pop out if you bear down gently, use a very mild suppository.

Faceplate Water Absorption

The wax-like faceplate of a colostomy bag is fine if you shower or swim. Because you only spend a short time showering and it doesn't absorb water fast, and if you take a swim, as long as you don't frolic in the pool for longer than half-an-hour or so, it will not absorb water and lift from your abdomen. The bag itself is waterproof.

When the faceplate absorbs moisture, it swells, becomes a pale white, and begins to lift off from where it has been attached on the stoma. The absorption starts at the edge and slowly, the wax starts to soften, becoming almost putty-like. Eventually, it spreads in towards the centre while losing its stickiness. At this point, the faceplate and bag start to come off, or, the plate will start to form loose pockets.

How can you avoid this from happening? Swim for no longer than 45 minutes and ensure you change the whole bag if it is a disposable colostomy bag, or the face-plate piece if it is a 2-piece system.

Pancaking (or Patty-caking)

This is an occurrence that many ostomates don't see as a problem, but it is an annoying one nonetheless. It's called pancaking or patty-caking. It occurs when stool collects around the stoma instead of going right into the colostomy bag. This stool forms a 'cake', the shape of a pancake and thickens around the stoma, pushing its way underneath the flange or faceplate as it accumulates.

This can cause irritation problems if you are sore around the stoma and may cause an infection. Pancaking also causes unpleasant odour or leaks as it pushes and lifts part of the flange off from the abdomen.

But why does pancaking occur?

It is caused by one of two things. It is either your stool has a sticky or thick consistency, or the appliance's filter is over-effective, meaning it lets out gas too quickly, causing the bag to lay like it is ironed flat against the abdomen. This problem can be tricky to resolve, but here are the ways I was able to resolve my pancaking issues whenever it occurs.

- I increased my fluid intake: This is the #1 remedy and it is important because if you drink enough fluids, preferably water, your waste will not become hard or sticky.
- Alter your diet slightly: Do this by increasing your fibre intake. This will help to alter the consistency of your stool.
- Blow a bit of air into the colostomy bag: Before fitting on your appliance, blow some air into your bag. This helps to prevent it from flattening against your tummy.
- Use filter stickers: Sometimes, the filter system can be over-effective so to avoid this, place a sticker (round white stickers that come with your *colostomy supplies*) over the filter hole. This way, the bag doesn't look 'sucked-up' and it will allow the gas that

precedes stooling create more space for the stool to move freely down the bag.

Remember that your stoma is like an alien stuck to your abdomen and needs extra care and attention if you wish to avoid (or keep to the barest minimum) unforeseen situations or colostomy bag mishaps.

Bag 'Blowouts'

Some colostomy problems and incidences are unavoidable. This is one of the troubling issues that I encountered now and then, but not that often. The term 'blowout' may sound like a disaster, but that's not the case. When it occurs, the colostomy pouch does not blow off like a burst balloon, splattering faeces all over the place. Rather, what happens is that for some reasons, the bag's waxy faceplate begins to flex and gradually lifts off from around the stoma.

So, what causes the plate to flex? It mostly has to do with the stoma but also has to do with stool consistency, lotions, and face-plate holes.

- **Stoma shrinkage**: In this instance, the stoma may shrink, for instance, when the weather is extremely cold.
- **Recede**: A receding stoma is one that is almost completely retracted into my body.
- **Lightly expand**: Sometimes, when the weather is extremely hot, or you've just had a hot bath or shower, the stoma expands a bit.
- **Be prolapsed**: Some stomas prolapse, and this can facilitate blowouts. A prolapse occurs when the bowel protrudes through the stoma opening in the stomach to a greater extent than was anticipated. A protruding bowel can vary from 2cm to 3cm, and sometimes as much as 10cm.

- **React to heat or cold**: The stoma sometimes shrinks, recedes, or lightly expands with excessive heat or intense cold.
- **Stool consistency**: Hard stool caused by constipation may not expel into the colostomy bag and will put some pressure on the rim of the cut face-plate holes
- **Faceplate-hole size**: A hole that's cut too large that doesn't fit snugly around the stoma leaves room for leakage and a slow but gradual lift of the faceplate.
- **Creams and lotions**: If the skin around the stoma is oily from the use of creams or oil the faceplate will not stick firmly on the abdomen and will lift off.

As the faceplate's lift widens, more stool seeps into these gaps. This is when leakages begin to occur. Eventually, the consistent leak causes the accumulation of waste which then blows-open a section of the waxy plate. Bag blow-outs can turn into a nasty situation if not remedied immediately.

Tell-tale signs of an impending bag blowout? Well, if you are perceptive, you will feel it coming on. You will experience a slight feeling of air pockets developing around your stoma and a horrifying warm feeling of the first faeces leak. About a second later, you will smell a faint (at first; it gets worse) whiff of stool coming from your abdominal area. This is usually the first sign of what may eventually result in a colostomy pouch blow-out.

What to do? Find a toilet and change your stoma bag. If you don't, though it happens slowly; gradually forming a "caking" around the stoma, it will eventually have an opening that will expand enough to leak faeces onto your clothing, and that will be so very unpleasant and, you will be the first person to perceive that whiff of odour. Don't dismiss it because it will only get worse. That first whiff of odour. is the main thing to look out for. Also, if you feel the slightest flexing of your faceplate along your skin folds, it's coming on.

When any of these happen, then you know it is time for a change. Also, avoid being caught unawares; always remember to carry spare colostomy bags along with you whenever you are away from home because blowouts" may occur, even if your colostomy bag is partially empty.

To manage this colostomy bag problem, all that's required is the replacement. However, after removing the offending appliance and wearing a fresh new one, you must clean the stoma and its surrounding area gently, including where the caking may have occurred. After I found ways to manage this problem, I rarely experienced it. These are the measures I took:

- I ensured that the skin area around my stoma is free from dirt, cream, or oil so that the faceplate can adhere firmly to my abdomen.
- I ate the right foods and stayed away from foods that make me constipated.
- I used modern colostomy bags which helped me manage colostomy bag problems with ease.
- I ensured that the cut-out stoma holes on the colostomy bag's waxy face-plate were the right size for my stoma.
- I rarely used pre-cut plates. They just never seemed to fit well around my stoma. There is an advantage in using modern pouches that you can cut yourself as the stoma sometimes changes in size.
- If the hole is remotely larger than the stoma, caking, and eventually colostomy bag blowouts may occur, and if too small, it will bruise the stoma and cause slight bleeding.
- If I can't resist eating food that's associated with constipation, I eat them only when I know I'll be staying home, like over the weekends.

Finally, depending on how long you'll be away from home, whether it is a couple of hours or the whole day, never have less than two to four spares colostomy bags with you.

Colostomy Reversal One Year After

My colostomy reversal procedure was done one year after my colostomy surgery. But what do you need to know about and stoma reversals and how long should you wait before the stoma reconnect procedure? Find out what to expect, and more.

My colostomy reversal procedure was exactly one year to the day that I had surgery for a temporary colostomy. When I had the ostomy, my doctor had advised that I'd have to wait a year for my stoma reconnect because my colon needed ample time to regenerate and heal completely. It was a process he always applied and because I had explicit trust in him, I was okay with his advice. He doesn't like to rush it.

And so, it was. Twelve months later, I had my temporary colostomy reversed; a colostomy take-down. With this reversal, my stoma was no longer necessary. It was pushed back in to reconnect it to my digestive tract and then was sealed up.

Not all colostomies can be reversed. The procedure to reverse your stoma is usually less demanding than the original stoma surgery, depending on whether you have any other medical complications or not. But your bowel and anal muscles must be working well for a successful reversal.

Additionally, the body must be well healed to undergo another operation. Your surgeon will not carry out a stoma reversal unless you are in good health, and not until you have fully recovered from the effects of the colostomy operation.

When a colostomy is reversible, the reasons could be that:

- Trauma and its subsequent damage to the abdomen and the colon are not critical.
- The damage to the colon is minimal.

- The colon has healed completely and can now be reconnected back.
- A colon cancer patient has healed well enough after the initial surgery and has fully recovered from other treatments like chemotherapy or radiotherapy.

The stoma-reconnect procedure is simpler and relatively straightforward and can take any time from sixty minutes to a couple of hours, depending on the complexity of the initial procedure. In my case, it took around an hour and forty-five minutes to reverse my colostomy.

The waiting period between the first procedure and its reversal is at the sole discretion of your doctor and can vary from a couple of months to a few years. As a surgeon, he or she is always in a better position to advise you as to when your stoma reversal will be carried out.

After my colon had sufficiently healed to my doctor's satisfaction, it was time for my procedure, and it was done by the same surgeon that performed the first operation. You may find that in most cases, it is the doctor that performed the initial surgery that will carry out a colostomy reversal, and more likely than not, performed at the same hospital.

My temporary colostomy was reversed by the same surgeon and I was attended to by the same Stoma Nurse.

The procedure simply involves pushing the stoma back in and reconnecting the healed colon to it (your digestive tract), using sutures that will dissolve in the body within three months or thereabouts. The reconnection allows the digestive tract to function as it did before colostomy surgery was carried out.

Most ostomy patients are well enough to leave the hospital within 4 to 8 days. I spent 9 days, simply because it took a bit longer for my bowel to start to function again, but it may take less time for some patients and a bit more for others.

The stoma position on the abdomen is stitched shut with either dissolvable sutures, or small metal staples that are eventually removed after complete healing of the spot which took mine about two weeks. Removal of stitches or staples will be carried out in the outpatient department of your hospital.

After my stoma reversal, I was able to eliminate faeces through my rectum though it took a short while. Initially, I had some light constipation, but it soon became functional. Some patients' experience the reverse and expel loose stool which may be frequent, but with time, the body and its digestive system settle back to normal.

My initial diet after my stoma reconnect consisted of light foods in small portions, but gradually, I reverted to my regular diet but still ate in moderation.

How Long Does It Take to Fully Recover?

It may take several weeks for a patient to recover from colostomy reversal surgery and return to normal daily activities. Though it usually takes between four to six weeks for most, the recovery time will depend on the type of operation initially performed; ascending, transverse, or descending colostomy.

Recovery time also depends on whether you have other medical conditions, your will and determination, your general attitude, and whether or not you develop post-surgery complications.

Post-Surgery Monitoring

I was checked and monitored constantly for any signs or symptoms of complications, and closely observed for signs of infection, which may indicate an internal leak of waste into the stomach. Tests were carried out frequently to ensure my recovery is normal and acceptable, and there were also very frequent checks on vital signs.

Recent Studies on Temporary Colostomy Patients

Latest research studies by the *University of Michigan Health System* tells us that temporary colostomy patients are generally not as accepting and happy as patients with a permanent colostomy. Strange, but true.

They say that patients with a temporary colostomy will always hope and yearn for a life without a colostomy. It is said that many may put their life on hold and may postpone getting on with their normal lifestyle and habits until their colostomies are reversed. On the other hand, ostomy patients with permanent colostomies soon adjust to their medical condition and quickly realise that there is no changing the fact that they'll live with a stoma for the rest of their lives. So, they deal with it squarely and move on happily with their lives.

For the temporary colostomy patient, a stoma reversal is a joy. I was happy it was all over. No more colostomy appliances, no more noisy wind, no more bag ballooning, and no more disposing of, or emptying faeces from colostomy bags.

My Inspiration

This awesome book - "I'd Like to Buy a Bowel Please" - that I purchased a few weeks after my surgical procedure gave me a glimpse into the daily challenges to expect as a colostomy patient. What I loved most about this book was the incredible spirit and sarcastic humour woven into it, with examples from ostomates on how they coped and soon moved on with their lives.

The author's wit was a great inspiration to me and I'm sure it will be for many others living with a temporary or permanent colostomy.

www.ingramcontent.com/pod-product-compliance
Lightning Source LLC
Chambersburg PA
CBHW070242220526
45465CB00004B/1495